THIS PLANNER
Belongs To:

_____

I'm PREGNANT!

HOW I FOUND OUT

MY REACTION

DUE DATE

WHAT I AM MOST EXCITED ABOUT

WHO I TOLD FIRST

WHAT I WANT YOU TO KNOW

MY BIRTH PLAN *Ideas*

WHO I WANT IN THE DELIVERY ROOM:

TYPE OF BIRTH

☐ VAGINAL ☐ WATER BIRTH

☐ C-SECTION ☐ VBAC

THOUGHTS ABOUT BIRTH AND WHAT IS MOST IMPORTANT TO ME

GETTING READY FOR THE BIG DAY: TO DO

NOTES & IDEAS (lighting, music, etc.)

40 Weeks

PREGNANCY Tracker

Keep track of how you're feeling every week of your pregnancy.

APPOINTMENT Tracker

Keep track of your pre-natal classes and doctor appointments.

DATE	TIME	ADDRESS	PURPOSE

BABY SHOPPING *List*

Start planning for the arrival of your baby by using the shopping list below.

Undershirts	Crib	Bottles
Socks	Bassinet	Bottle Liners
Pajamas	Baby Bath tub	Nursing Bra & Pads
Sweaters	Car Seat	Breast Pump
Onesies	Stroller	Formula
Hats	High Chair	Pacifiers
Bibs	Play Pen	Bottle Brush
Blanket	Baby Swing	Burp Cloths
Diaper Bag	Monitor	Bottle Sanitizer
Mitts	Change Table	Nipples
Diapers	Rocking Chair	Baby Powder
Booties	Night Light	Baby Wipes
Receiving Blankets	Mobile	
Crib Sheet	Bouncer	
Wash Cloths	Nail Clippers	
Towels	Teething Toys	
	Baby Wipes	
	Diaper Pail	

PREGNANCY *Tracker*

 Weight Tracker Chart

It's important to keep track of your weight throughout your pregnancy.
Record your weight in the chart below every week, starting at week 4.

WEEKLY WEIGHT TRACKER									
4		12		20		28		36	
5		13		21		29		37	
6		14		22		30		38	
7		15		23		31		39	
8		16		24		32		40	
9		17		25		33			
10		18		26		34			
11		19		27		35			

 NOTE — According to the American Pregnancy Association, pregnant women should consume up to 300 more calories a day. Further, healthy eating is critical to your baby's development which means you should make sure to maintain a well-balanced diet, high in nutrients and proteins.

HEALTHY FOOD *Ideas*

VEGETABLES & LOW SUGAR FRUIT	PROTEINS	COMPLEX CARBS	HEALTHY FATS	SUPPLEMENTS
Leafy greens (spinach, etc.)	Organic meat	Beets	Avocado	Vitamin D
Broccoli	Liver	Carrots	Olive Oil	Fish Oil
Cauliflower	Bone Broth	Sweet Potatoes	Coconut Oil	Algae Oil
Cabbage	Beans	Yams	Yogurt	Probiotics
Asparagus	Lentils	Parsnips	Almonds	Ginger Pills
Cucumber	Flax Seed	Turnips	Mixed Nuts	Licorice Root
Mushrooms	Pumpkin Seed	Pumpkin	Soybean	Magnesium
Celery	Chia Seed	Buckwheat	Olives	Krill Oil
Radish	Salmon	Brown Rice	Nut butter	Iron Pills
Grapefruit & Melon	Herring	Squash		
Berries (all kinds)				
Peaches (with skin)				

Tracker — PRE-NATAL Visits

Important Dates

Keep track of your pre-natal appointments and include a summary of each visit.

DATE	
HOW FAR ALONG?	
YOUR WEIGHT	
BLOOD PRESSURE	
FETAL HEART RATE	
DOCTOR	

SUMMARY OF APPOINTMENT

NOTES:

NEXT APPOINTMENT.:

DATE	
HOW FAR ALONG?	
YOUR WEIGHT	
BLOOD PRESSURE	
FETAL HEART RATE	
DOCTOR	

SUMMARY OF APPOINTMENT

NOTES:

NEXT APPOINTMENT.:

DATE	
HOW FAR ALONG?	
YOUR WEIGHT	
BLOOD PRESSURE	
FETAL HEART RATE	
DOCTOR	

SUMMARY OF APPOINTMENT

NOTES:

NEXT APPOINTMENT.:

1-13 Weeks

FIRST Trimester

Journal your thoughts and feelings during each trimester so you can later reflect on your pregnancy journey.

HOW I FELT DURING MY FIRST TRIMESTER

MY FAVORITE MEMORIES

SYMPTOMS & CRAVINGS

ENERGY
♥ ♥ ♥ ♥ ♥ ♥

SLEEP
♥ ♥ ♥ ♥ ♥ ♥

CRAVINGS
♥ ♥ ♥ ♥ ♥ ♥

MOODS
♥ ♥ ♥ ♥ ♥ ♥

TO DO LIST: 1st TRIMESTER

FIRST TRIMESTER *Photos*

MEMORIES ARE FOREVER

SECOND *Trimester*

14-27 Weeks

HOW I FELT DURING MY SECOND TRIMESTER

MY FAVORITE MEMORIES

SYMPTOMS & CRAVINGS

ENERGY
♥ ♥ ♥ ♥ ♥ ♥

SLEEP
♥ ♥ ♥ ♥ ♥ ♥

CRAVINGS
♥ ♥ ♥ ♥ ♥ ♥

MOODS
♥ ♥ ♥ ♥ ♥ ♥

TO DO LIST: 2nd TRIMESTER

SECOND TRIMESTER *Photos*

MEMORIES ARE FOREVER

THIRD Trimester

28-40 Weeks

HOW I FELT DURING MY THIRD TRIMESTER

MY FAVORITE MEMORIES

SYMPTOMS & CRAVINGS

ENERGY
♥ ♥ ♥ ♥ ♥ ♥

SLEEP
♥ ♥ ♥ ♥ ♥ ♥

CRAVINGS
♥ ♥ ♥ ♥ ♥ ♥

MOODS
♥ ♥ ♥ ♥ ♥ ♥

TO DO LIST: 3rd TRIMESTER

THIRD TRIMESTER *Photos*

MEMORIES ARE FOREVER

MY BABY Shower

BABY SHOWER PHOTOS

GAMES PLAYED

ON THE MENU

HIGHLIGHTS & MEMORIES

MY BABY *Shower Gifts*

Keep track of your baby shower gifts and send thank you notes

NAME	GIFT	ADDRESS	SENT?

NURSERY *Planner*

COLOR SCHEME IDEAS:			

ITEM TO PURCHASE	PRICE	NOTES

FURNITURE IDEAS

DECORATIVE IDEAS

BABY NAME *Ideas*

TOP 3 BOY NAMES

NAME MEANINGS

TOP 3 GIRL NAMES

NAME MEANINGS

BABY NAME RESOURCES (LIST YOUR FAVORITE PARENTING & PREGNANCY WEBSITES):		

OTHER BOY NAME POSSIBILITIES	OTHER GIRL NAME POSSIBILITES

HOSPITAL *Checklist*

FOR ME	FOR PARTNER	FOR BABY

PREGNANCY SHOPPING List

BABY CLOTHING	SUPPLIES/MEDICATION	FURNITURE/TOYS

FIRST TRIMESTER SHOPPING	SECOND TRIMESTER SHOPPING	THIRD TRIMESTER SHOPPING

Tracker: FETAL Movement

Starting around week 16, keep track of when you feel your baby move.

WEEK 16	TIME	NOTES
MON		
TUE		
WED		
THU		
FRI		
SAT		
SUN		

WEEK 17	TIME	NOTES
MON		
TUE		
WED		
THU		
FRI		
SAT		
SUN		

WEEK 18	TIME	NOTES
MON		
TUE		
WED		
THU		
FRI		
SAT		
SUN		

WEEK 19	TIME	NOTES
MON		
TUE		
WED		
THU		
FRI		
SAT		
SUN		

WEEK 20	TIME	NOTES
MON		
TUE		
WED		
THU		
FRI		
SAT		
SUN		

WEEK 21	TIME	NOTES
MON		
TUE		
WED		
THU		
FRI		
SAT		
SUN		

WEEK 22	TIME	NOTES
MON		
TUE		
WED		
THU		
FRI		
SAT		
SUN		

WEEK 23	TIME	NOTES
MON		
TUE		
WED		
THU		
FRI		
SAT		
SUN		

WEEK 24	TIME	NOTES
MON		
TUE		
WED		
THU		
FRI		
SAT		
SUN		

Tracker: FETAL Movement

WEEK 25	TIME	NOTES
MON		
TUE		
WED		
THU		
FRI		
SAT		
SUN		

WEEK 26	TIME	NOTES
MON		
TUE		
WED		
THU		
FRI		
SAT		
SUN		

WEEK 27	TIME	NOTES
MON		
TUE		
WED		
THU		
FRI		
SAT		
SUN		

WEEK 28	TIME	NOTES
MON		
TUE		
WED		
THU		
FRI		
SAT		
SUN		

WEEK 29	TIME	NOTES
MON		
TUE		
WED		
THU		
FRI		
SAT		
SUN		

WEEK 30	TIME	NOTES
MON		
TUE		
WED		
THU		
FRI		
SAT		
SUN		

WEEK 31	TIME	NOTES
MON		
TUE		
WED		
THU		
FRI		
SAT		
SUN		

WEEK 32	TIME	NOTES
MON		
TUE		
WED		
THU		
FRI		
SAT		
SUN		

WEEK 33	TIME	NOTES
MON		
TUE		
WED		
THU		
FRI		
SAT		
SUN		

Tracker FETAL Movement

WEEK 34	TIME	NOTES
MON		
TUE		
WED		
THU		
FRI		
SAT		
SUN		

WEEK 35	TIME	NOTES
MON		
TUE		
WED		
THU		
FRI		
SAT		
SUN		

WEEK 36	TIME	NOTES
MON		
TUE		
WED		
THU		
FRI		
SAT		
SUN		

WEEK 37	TIME	NOTES
MON		
TUE		
WED		
THU		
FRI		
SAT		
SUN		

WEEK 38	TIME	NOTES
MON		
TUE		
WED		
THU		
FRI		
SAT		
SUN		

WEEK 39	TIME	NOTES
MON		
TUE		
WED		
THU		
FRI		
SAT		
SUN		

WEEK 40	TIME	NOTES
MON		
TUE		
WED		
THU		
FRI		
SAT		
SUN		

NOTES

Week 4

PREGNANCY *Journal*

Your baby is the size of a poppy seed!

TOTAL WEIGHT GAIN

BELLY MEASUREMENT

BABY BUMP PHOTO

WEEKLY REFLECTIONS

SYMPTOMS & CRAVINGS

WHAT I WANT TO REMEMBER MOST

I'M MOST EXCITED ABOUT

I'M MOST NERVOUS ABOUT

Dear Baby,

Dear Baby

PREGNANCY *Journal*

TODAY'S DATE

WEEKS PREGNANT

HOW I'M FEELING TODAY

What I want you to know

Week 5

PREGNANCY *Journal*

Your baby is the size of a peppercorn!

TOTAL WEIGHT GAIN

BELLY MEASUREMENT

BABY BUMP PHOTO

WEEKLY REFLECTIONS

SYMPTOMS & CRAVINGS

WHAT I WANT TO REMEMBER MOST

I'M MOST EXCITED ABOUT

I'M MOST NERVOUS ABOUT

Dear Baby,

Dear Baby

PREGNANCY *Journal*

TODAY'S DATE

WEEKS PREGNANT

HOW I'M FEELING TODAY

What I want you to know

Week 6

PREGNANCY Journal

Your baby is the size of a sweet pea!

TOTAL WEIGHT GAIN

BELLY MEASUREMENT

BABY BUMP PHOTO

WEEKLY REFLECTIONS

SYMPTOMS & CRAVINGS

WHAT I WANT TO REMEMBER MOST

I'M MOST EXCITED ABOUT

I'M MOST NERVOUS ABOUT

Dear Baby,

PREGNANCY *Journal*

TODAY'S DATE

WEEKS PREGNANT

HOW I'M FEELING TODAY

What I want you to know

PREGNANCY *Journal*

Week 7

Your baby is the size of a blueberry!

TOTAL WEIGHT GAIN

BELLY MEASUREMENT

BABY BUMP PHOTO

WEEKLY REFLECTIONS

SYMPTOMS & CRAVINGS

WHAT I WANT TO REMEMBER MOST

I'M MOST EXCITED ABOUT

I'M MOST NERVOUS ABOUT

Dear Baby,

Dear Baby
PREGNANCY *Journal*

TODAY'S DATE

WEEKS PREGNANT

HOW I'M FEELING TODAY

What I want you to know

Week 8 — PREGNANCY Journal

Your baby is the size of a raspberry!

TOTAL WEIGHT GAIN

BELLY MEASUREMENT

BABY BUMP PHOTO

WEEKLY REFLECTIONS

SYMPTOMS & CRAVINGS

WHAT I WANT TO REMEMBER MOST

I'M MOST EXCITED ABOUT

I'M MOST NERVOUS ABOUT

Dear Baby,

PREGNANCY *Journal*

TODAY'S DATE

WEEKS PREGNANT

HOW I'M FEELING TODAY

What I want you to know

PREGNANCY Journal

Week 9

Your baby is the size of a grape!

TOTAL WEIGHT GAIN

BELLY MEASUREMENT

BABY BUMP PHOTO

WEEKLY REFLECTIONS

SYMPTOMS & CRAVINGS

WHAT I WANT TO REMEMBER MOST

I'M MOST EXCITED ABOUT

I'M MOST NERVOUS ABOUT

Dear Baby,

PREGNANCY *Journal*

Dear Baby

TODAY'S DATE

WEEKS PREGNANT

HOW I'M FEELING TODAY

What I want you to know

PREGNANCY *Journal*

Week 10

Your baby is the size of a prune!

TOTAL WEIGHT GAIN

BELLY MEASUREMENT

BABY BUMP PHOTO

WEEKLY REFLECTIONS

SYMPTOMS & CRAVINGS

WHAT I WANT TO REMEMBER MOST

I'M MOST EXCITED ABOUT

I'M MOST NERVOUS ABOUT

Dear Baby,

PREGNANCY *Journal*

TODAY'S DATE

WEEKS PREGNANT

HOW I'M FEELING TODAY

What I want you to know

Week 11

PREGNANCY *Journal*

Your baby is the size of a lime!

TOTAL WEIGHT GAIN

BELLY MEASUREMENT

BABY BUMP PHOTO

WEEKLY REFLECTIONS

SYMPTOMS & CRAVINGS

WHAT I WANT TO REMEMBER MOST

I'M MOST EXCITED ABOUT

I'M MOST NERVOUS ABOUT

Dear Baby,

PREGNANCY *Journal*

TODAY'S DATE

WEEKS PREGNANT

HOW I'M FEELING TODAY

What I want you to know

Week 12

PREGNANCY *Journal*

Your baby is the size of a plum!

TOTAL WEIGHT GAIN

BELLY MEASUREMENT

BABY BUMP PHOTO

WEEKLY REFLECTIONS

SYMPTOMS & CRAVINGS

WHAT I WANT TO REMEMBER MOST

I'M MOST EXCITED ABOUT

I'M MOST NERVOUS ABOUT

Dear Baby,

ULTRASOUND Scan

ULTRASOUND PHOTO

ULTRASOUND RESULTS

BABY'S LENGTH:

BABY'S WEIGHT:

BPD:

DUE DATE:

Notes

PREGNANCY *Journal*

TODAY'S DATE

WEEKS PREGNANT

HOW I'M FEELING TODAY

―― *What I want you to know* ――

PREGNANCY *Journal*

Week 13

Your baby is the size of a peach!

TOTAL WEIGHT GAIN

BELLY MEASUREMENT

BABY BUMP PHOTO

WEEKLY REFLECTIONS

SYMPTOMS & CRAVINGS

WHAT I WANT TO REMEMBER MOST

I'M MOST EXCITED ABOUT

I'M MOST NERVOUS ABOUT

Dear Baby,

PREGNANCY *Journal*

Dear Baby

TODAY'S DATE

WEEKS PREGNANT

HOW I'M FEELING TODAY

What I want you to know

PREGNANCY *Journal*

Week 14

Your baby is the size of a lemon!

TOTAL WEIGHT GAIN

BELLY MEASUREMENT

BABY BUMP PHOTO

WEEKLY REFLECTIONS

SYMPTOMS & CRAVINGS

WHAT I WANT TO REMEMBER MOST

I'M MOST EXCITED ABOUT

I'M MOST NERVOUS ABOUT

Dear Baby,

PREGNANCY *Journal*

TODAY'S DATE

WEEKS PREGNANT

HOW I'M FEELING TODAY

What I want you to know

Week 15

PREGNANCY *Journal*

Your baby is the size of an apple!

TOTAL WEIGHT GAIN

BELLY MEASUREMENT

BABY BUMP PHOTO

WEEKLY REFLECTIONS

SYMPTOMS & CRAVINGS

WHAT I WANT TO REMEMBER MOST

I'M MOST EXCITED ABOUT

I'M MOST NERVOUS ABOUT

Dear Baby,

PREGNANCY *Journal*

TODAY'S DATE

WEEKS PREGNANT

HOW I'M FEELING TODAY

What I want you to know

Week 16 | PREGNANCY *Journal*

Your baby is the size of an avocado!

TOTAL WEIGHT GAIN

BELLY MEASUREMENT

BABY BUMP PHOTO

WEEKLY REFLECTIONS

SYMPTOMS & CRAVINGS

WHAT I WANT TO REMEMBER MOST

I'M MOST EXCITED ABOUT

I'M MOST NERVOUS ABOUT

Dear Baby,

Dear Baby

PREGNANCY *Journal*

TODAY'S DATE

WEEKS PREGNANT

HOW I'M FEELING TODAY

What I want you to know

PREGNANCY *Journal*

Week 17

Your baby is the size of a pear!

TOTAL WEIGHT GAIN

BELLY MEASUREMENT

BABY BUMP PHOTO

WEEKLY REFLECTIONS

SYMPTOMS & CRAVINGS

WHAT I WANT TO REMEMBER MOST

I'M MOST EXCITED ABOUT

I'M MOST NERVOUS ABOUT

Dear Baby,

PREGNANCY *Journal*

TODAY'S DATE

WEEKS PREGNANT

HOW I'M FEELING TODAY

What I want you to know

PREGNANCY *Journal*

Week 18

Your baby is the size of a sweet potato!

TOTAL WEIGHT GAIN

BELLY MEASUREMENT

BABY BUMP PHOTO

WEEKLY REFLECTIONS

SYMPTOMS & CRAVINGS

WHAT I WANT TO REMEMBER MOST

I'M MOST EXCITED ABOUT

I'M MOST NERVOUS ABOUT

Dear Baby,

Dear Baby

PREGNANCY *Journal*

TODAY'S DATE

WEEKS PREGNANT

HOW I'M FEELING TODAY

What I want you to know

Week 19 — PREGNANCY Journal

Your baby is the size of a mango!

TOTAL WEIGHT GAIN

BELLY MEASUREMENT

BABY BUMP PHOTO

WEEKLY REFLECTIONS

SYMPTOMS & CRAVINGS

WHAT I WANT TO REMEMBER MOST

I'M MOST EXCITED ABOUT

I'M MOST NERVOUS ABOUT

Dear Baby,

Dear Baby — PREGNANCY *Journal*

TODAY'S DATE

WEEKS PREGNANT

HOW I'M FEELING TODAY

What I want you to know

PREGNANCY *Journal*

Week 20

Your baby is the size of a banana!

TOTAL WEIGHT GAIN

BELLY MEASUREMENT

BABY BUMP PHOTO

WEEKLY REFLECTIONS

SYMPTOMS & CRAVINGS

WHAT I WANT TO REMEMBER MOST

I'M MOST EXCITED ABOUT

I'M MOST NERVOUS ABOUT

Dear Baby,

ULTRASOUND Scan

ULTRASOUND PHOTO

ULTRASOUND RESULTS

BABY'S LENGTH:

BABY'S WEIGHT:

BPD:

DUE DATE:

Notes

PREGNANCY *Journal*

TODAY'S DATE

WEEKS PREGNANT

HOW I'M FEELING TODAY

What I want you to know

Week 21

PREGNANCY *Journal*

Your baby is the size of a carrot!

TOTAL WEIGHT GAIN

BELLY MEASUREMENT

BABY BUMP PHOTO

WEEKLY REFLECTIONS

SYMPTOMS & CRAVINGS

WHAT I WANT TO REMEMBER MOST

I'M MOST EXCITED ABOUT

I'M MOST NERVOUS ABOUT

Dear Baby,

PREGNANCY *Journal*

TODAY'S DATE

WEEKS PREGNANT

HOW I'M FEELING TODAY

What I want you to know

PREGNANCY *Journal*

Week 22

Your baby is the size of a papaya!

TOTAL WEIGHT GAIN

BELLY MEASUREMENT

BABY BUMP PHOTO

WEEKLY REFLECTIONS

SYMPTOMS & CRAVINGS

WHAT I WANT TO REMEMBER MOST

I'M MOST EXCITED ABOUT

I'M MOST NERVOUS ABOUT

Dear Baby,

PREGNANCY *Journal*

TODAY'S DATE

WEEKS PREGNANT

HOW I'M FEELING TODAY

What I want you to know

PREGNANCY *Journal*

Week 23

Your baby is the size of a grapefruit!

TOTAL WEIGHT GAIN

BELLY MEASUREMENT

BABY BUMP PHOTO

WEEKLY REFLECTIONS

SYMPTOMS & CRAVINGS

WHAT I WANT TO REMEMBER MOST

I'M MOST EXCITED ABOUT

I'M MOST NERVOUS ABOUT

Dear Baby,

PREGNANCY *Journal*

TODAY'S DATE

WEEKS PREGNANT

HOW I'M FEELING TODAY

What I want you to know

PREGNANCY Journal

Week 24

Your baby is the size of a cantaloupe!

TOTAL WEIGHT GAIN

BELLY MEASUREMENT

BABY BUMP PHOTO

WEEKLY REFLECTIONS

SYMPTOMS & CRAVINGS

WHAT I WANT TO REMEMBER MOST

I'M MOST EXCITED ABOUT

I'M MOST NERVOUS ABOUT

Dear Baby,

PREGNANCY *Journal*

TODAY'S DATE

WEEKS PREGNANT

HOW I'M FEELING TODAY

What I want you to know

PREGNANCY *Journal*

Week 25

Your baby is the size of a cauliflower!

TOTAL WEIGHT GAIN

BELLY MEASUREMENT

BABY BUMP PHOTO

WEEKLY REFLECTIONS

SYMPTOMS & CRAVINGS

WHAT I WANT TO REMEMBER MOST

I'M MOST EXCITED ABOUT

I'M MOST NERVOUS ABOUT

Dear Baby,

PREGNANCY *Journal*

TODAY'S DATE

WEEKS PREGNANT

HOW I'M FEELING TODAY

What I want you to know

PREGNANCY *Journal*

Week 26

Your baby is the size of a head of lettuce!

TOTAL WEIGHT GAIN

BELLY MEASUREMENT

BABY BUMP PHOTO

WEEKLY REFLECTIONS

SYMPTOMS & CRAVINGS

WHAT I WANT TO REMEMBER MOST

I'M MOST EXCITED ABOUT

I'M MOST NERVOUS ABOUT

Dear Baby,

PREGNANCY *Journal*

TODAY'S DATE

WEEKS PREGNANT

HOW I'M FEELING TODAY

What I want you to know

PREGNANCY *Journal*

Week 27

Your baby is the size of a rutabaga!

TOTAL WEIGHT GAIN

BELLY MEASUREMENT

BABY BUMP PHOTO

WEEKLY REFLECTIONS

SYMPTOMS & CRAVINGS

WHAT I WANT TO REMEMBER MOST

I'M MOST EXCITED ABOUT

I'M MOST NERVOUS ABOUT

Dear Baby,

Dear Baby

PREGNANCY *Journal*

♥♥♥♥♥♥♥♥♥♥♥♥♥♥♥♥♥♥♥

TODAY'S DATE

WEEKS PREGNANT

HOW I'M FEELING TODAY

―― *What I want you to know* ――

PREGNANCY *Journal*

Week 28

Your baby is the size of an eggplant!

TOTAL WEIGHT GAIN

BELLY MEASUREMENT

BABY BUMP PHOTO

WEEKLY REFLECTIONS

SYMPTOMS & CRAVINGS

WHAT I WANT TO REMEMBER MOST

I'M MOST EXCITED ABOUT

I'M MOST NERVOUS ABOUT

Dear Baby,

PREGNANCY *Journal*

TODAY'S DATE

WEEKS PREGNANT

HOW I'M FEELING TODAY

What I want you to know

PREGNANCY Journal

Week 29

Your baby is the size of an acorn squash!

TOTAL WEIGHT GAIN

BELLY MEASUREMENT

BABY BUMP PHOTO

WEEKLY REFLECTIONS

SYMPTOMS & CRAVINGS

WHAT I WANT TO REMEMBER MOST

I'M MOST EXCITED ABOUT

I'M MOST NERVOUS ABOUT

Dear Baby,

PREGNANCY *Journal*

TODAY'S DATE

WEEKS PREGNANT

HOW I'M FEELING TODAY

What I want you to know

PREGNANCY *Journal*

Week 30

Your baby is the size of a cucumber!

TOTAL WEIGHT GAIN

BELLY MEASUREMENT

BABY BUMP PHOTO

WEEKLY REFLECTIONS

SYMPTOMS & CRAVINGS

WHAT I WANT TO REMEMBER MOST

I'M MOST EXCITED ABOUT

I'M MOST NERVOUS ABOUT

Dear Baby,

PREGNANCY *Journal*

TODAY'S DATE

WEEKS PREGNANT

HOW I'M FEELING TODAY

What I want you to know

Week 31 — PREGNANCY *Journal*

Your baby is the size of a pineapple!

TOTAL WEIGHT GAIN

BELLY MEASUREMENT

BABY BUMP PHOTO

WEEKLY REFLECTIONS

SYMPTOMS & CRAVINGS

WHAT I WANT TO REMEMBER MOST

I'M MOST EXCITED ABOUT

I'M MOST NERVOUS ABOUT

Dear Baby,

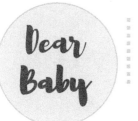

PREGNANCY *Journal*

TODAY'S DATE

WEEKS PREGNANT

HOW I'M FEELING TODAY

What I want you to know

PREGNANCY *Journal*

Week 32

Your baby is the size of a squash!

TOTAL WEIGHT GAIN

BELLY MEASUREMENT

BABY BUMP PHOTO

WEEKLY REFLECTIONS

SYMPTOMS & CRAVINGS

WHAT I WANT TO REMEMBER MOST

I'M MOST EXCITED ABOUT

I'M MOST NERVOUS ABOUT

Dear Baby,

PREGNANCY *Journal*

TODAY'S DATE

WEEKS PREGNANT

HOW I'M FEELING TODAY

What I want you to know

PREGNANCY *Journal*

Week 33

Your baby is the size of a durian!

TOTAL WEIGHT GAIN

BELLY MEASUREMENT

BABY BUMP PHOTO

WEEKLY REFLECTIONS

SYMPTOMS & CRAVINGS

WHAT I WANT TO REMEMBER MOST

I'M MOST EXCITED ABOUT

I'M MOST NERVOUS ABOUT

Dear Baby,

PREGNANCY *Journal*

TODAY'S DATE

WEEKS PREGNANT

HOW I'M FEELING TODAY

What I want you to know

PREGNANCY *Journal*

Week 34

Your baby is the size of a butternut squash!

TOTAL WEIGHT GAIN

BELLY MEASUREMENT

BABY BUMP PHOTO

WEEKLY REFLECTIONS

SYMPTOMS & CRAVINGS

WHAT I WANT TO REMEMBER MOST

I'M MOST EXCITED ABOUT

I'M MOST NERVOUS ABOUT

Dear Baby,

PREGNANCY *Journal*

TODAY'S DATE

WEEKS PREGNANT

HOW I'M FEELING TODAY

What I want you to know

Week 35

PREGNANCY *Journal*

Your baby is the size of a coconut!

TOTAL WEIGHT GAIN

BELLY MEASUREMENT

BABY BUMP PHOTO

WEEKLY REFLECTIONS

SYMPTOMS & CRAVINGS

WHAT I WANT TO REMEMBER MOST

I'M MOST EXCITED ABOUT

I'M MOST NERVOUS ABOUT

Dear Baby,

PREGNANCY *Journal*

TODAY'S DATE

WEEKS PREGNANT

HOW I'M FEELING TODAY

What I want you to know

Week 36

PREGNANCY *Journal*

Your baby is the size of a honeydew melon!

TOTAL WEIGHT GAIN

BELLY MEASUREMENT

BABY BUMP PHOTO

WEEKLY REFLECTIONS

SYMPTOMS & CRAVINGS

WHAT I WANT TO REMEMBER MOST

I'M MOST EXCITED ABOUT

I'M MOST NERVOUS ABOUT

Dear Baby,

PREGNANCY *Journal*

TODAY'S DATE

WEEKS PREGNANT

HOW I'M FEELING TODAY

What I want you to know

PREGNANCY *Journal*

Week 37

Your baby is the size of a Winter Melon!

TOTAL WEIGHT GAIN

BELLY MEASUREMENT

BABY BUMP PHOTO

WEEKLY REFLECTIONS

SYMPTOMS & CRAVINGS

WHAT I WANT TO REMEMBER MOST

I'M MOST EXCITED ABOUT

I'M MOST NERVOUS ABOUT

Dear Baby,

PREGNANCY *Journal*

TODAY'S DATE

WEEKS PREGNANT

HOW I'M FEELING TODAY

What I want you to know

PREGNANCY *Journal*

Week 38

Your baby is the size of a pumpkin!

TOTAL WEIGHT GAIN

BELLY MEASUREMENT

BABY BUMP PHOTO

WEEKLY REFLECTIONS

SYMPTOMS & CRAVINGS

WHAT I WANT TO REMEMBER MOST

I'M MOST EXCITED ABOUT

I'M MOST NERVOUS ABOUT

Dear Baby,

Dear Baby

PREGNANCY *Journal*

TODAY'S DATE

WEEKS PREGNANT

HOW I'M FEELING TODAY

What I want you to know

PREGNANCY *Journal*

Week 39

Your baby is the size of a watermelon!

TOTAL WEIGHT GAIN

BELLY MEASUREMENT

BABY BUMP PHOTO

WEEKLY REFLECTIONS

SYMPTOMS & CRAVINGS

WHAT I WANT TO REMEMBER MOST

I'M MOST EXCITED ABOUT

I'M MOST NERVOUS ABOUT

Dear Baby,

PREGNANCY *Journal*

TODAY'S DATE

WEEKS PREGNANT

HOW I'M FEELING TODAY

What I want you to know

Week 40

PREGNANCY *Journal*

Your baby is the size of a jack fruit!

TOTAL WEIGHT GAIN

BELLY MEASUREMENT

BABY BUMP PHOTO

WEEKLY REFLECTIONS

SYMPTOMS & CRAVINGS

WHAT I WANT TO REMEMBER MOST

I'M MOST EXCITED ABOUT

I'M MOST NERVOUS ABOUT

Dear Baby,

PREGNANCY *Journal*

TODAY'S DATE

WEEKS PREGNANT

HOW I'M FEELING TODAY

What I want you to know

Printed in Great Britain
by Amazon